Aromatherapy

How to use aromatherapy and essential oils, including aromatherapy cures, remedies, and more!

Table Of Contents

Introduction

I want to thank you and congratulate you for downloading the book, *"Aromatherapy"*.

This book contains helpful information about aromatherapy, and how you can begin to use aromatherapy and essential oils to improve your health!

You will soon learn about the different essential oils that you can use, what they can be used for, and also how to use them.

You will discover the different ways of blending and using oils, including the use of carrier and base oils.

This book will explain to you tips and techniques that will allow you to successfully use aromatherapy for a range of benefits, including health remedies, relaxation, lowering blood pressure, and more!

Whether you're new to aromatherapy, or have used it before, this book will have something to offer you and serve as a complete guide.

Thanks again for downloading this book, I hope you enjoy it!

Chapter 1: What Is Aromatherapy?

By now, you may already know about aromatherapy as well as some of the benefits it can provide you with. However, contrary to what most people believe, it isn't just about surrounding yourself with pleasant smells. Aromatherapy goes much deeper than that and if used correctly, can easily help your body as well as your mind heal.

In the most basic sense, aromatherapy is basically the practice of using plant oils, including some of the more popular essential oils, as a way of healing a person. It is no secret that essential oils, also known as the pure essence of the plant you extract it from, have many major health benefits.

It is considered to be a form of alternative medicine, a natural and holistic variety, which is great if you're looking for a safe way of healing yourself. What most people tend to misunderstand is the fact that it doesn't just involve inhaling the scent of a particular oil. Aromatherapy is actually a broader term which encompasses the different uses of oils. They can be applied to the body in the form of a topical remedy or through the most common use, inhalation.

So what's the science behind it?

Many believe that inhaling essential oils actually helps in stimulating certain parts of our brain through the olfactory system. This then sends a signal to the limbic system of our brain, the same part that controls our emotions as well as relives memories- often the ones we associate with feeling good. This is why many people who have tried aromatherapy claim that it makes them feel calm and relaxed. However, depending on the kind you use, it can also stimulate you and make you more alert.

Essential oils are also said to have a pharmacological effect while professional aromatherapists claim that it also involves a synergy between the oils and the human body. Regarding this, studies are still being conducted but as far as history goes - aromatherapy certainly works.

In France as well as most of Western Europe, it is actually incorporated into the mainstream medical field where it is often used as an antibacterial, antifungal, antiviral and antiseptic. Compare that to places such as the USA, UK and Canada where its effects are not recognized by the mainstream medical community and often relegated to a spot in the folk medicine category.

These are comprised of aromatic molecules which are, typically, readily absorbed through our skin or by breathing in. They then enter our bloodstream and be carried throughout our body where they can deliver their healing effects. Now, do keep in mind that the essential oils often used by aromatherapists are very concentrated and nothing like the cheap ones you can find for a few dollars in many home good stores.

This is where the difference lies.

It is important that you make use of high quality essential oils as these are the ones that carry the components you need to heal your body. The purer it is, the better the effects will be. You usually don't require a large amount of oil, often, a drop is more than enough. While they might cost more than your average essential oil, the benefits are certainly worth every penny - especially if you use them correctly.

A Holistic Approach:

Aromatherapy has been around for quite a while but the recent resurgence of its popularity can be attributed to the growing worldwide movement wherein people are choosing to go natural when it comes to the things they use on their body. It is for this reason that aromatherapy has become one of the most sought after complementary therapies and has been used for a variety of different health problems, treating both acute as well as chronic stages of illnesses.

The great thing about going natural for your health is that unlike chemical-based medicines, natural means you're not damaging any other part of your body. In fact, many natural remedies can help boost other aspects of your well-being such as your immune system. In other words, it is a more holistic approach to your health and recovery.

A professional aromatherapist would actually take into account your medical history, general health as well as lifestyle habits and even your emotional condition before starting you up on a treatment. This is because during the process itself, it isn't just your body that will experience healing - it can actually heal your mind as well and relieve other symptoms or issues that you might be experiencing. There's no risk of getting addicted to essential oils, quite unlike many other prescription medications.

Chapter 2: Aromatherapy Benefits

Essential oils have certainly secured their spot when it comes to an all-natural beauty routine. They are safe and chemical free alternatives to your more traditional cosmetics which can potentially contain harmful ingredients such as toxins. However, they can do more than just make you look and smell good. These essential oils, coupled with aromatherapy can actually help boost your overall well-being. Who wouldn't want to feel good from the inside out?

Here's how aromatherapy can benefit you:

- **Reduces stress significantly.**

One of the biggest enemies of good health is stress. You may not think much of it but dealing with a lot of stress can actually lead to you getting physically ill. However, the reality is that stress isn't something you can simply walk away from. This is especially the case if it's related to your work - you can't exactly quit, right? So what do you do? Pamper yourself every night after work. Bring out your aromatherapy kit and bask in the relaxing ambiance it creates. This is also great before bedtime as it will help you sleep better.

– **Fight the blues.**

You may not believe this but certain scents can effectively uplift your senses and in the process, your mood. This is why many people turn to aromatherapy when seeking to reduce the effects of depression or even simple melancholy blues. If you're feeling down in the dumps, getting a massage using aromatherapy has been shown to help improve your mood.

– **Relieving pain.**

Have you been exercising too much? Are your legs hurting from shopping all day or are you trying to get past menstrual pains? Well, aromatherapy can help relieve all of that and help you rest better. By calming your mind and stimulating the pressure sensors in your brain, aromatherapy can effectively help in reducing the amount of pain that you feel in an all-natural way. No more popping pills just to feel better!

– **Improve blood pressure.**

For patients with hypertension, aromatherapy can be used to lower blood pressure effectively and naturally. This occurs because the oils allow the body to relax, and subsequently your blood pressure begins to drop. After all, stress and anxiety can cause blood pressure levels to rise significantly. This can happen countless times a day and if you're not careful, can become a serious health issue as well. So avoid this and unwind through the use of aromatherapy whenever necessary.

Chapter 3: Best Essential Oils To Keep At Home

Now that we've established the fact that aromatherapy can help improve your health naturally, it's time we look at some of the common essential oils that can aid in making this happen. Different essential oils have differing effects on the body and as such, you want to familiarize yourself with some of them in order to make sure that you're using the right one for your needs.

In this list, we're including ones that have been used throughout history as a cure for just about anything. From skin problems such as acne to improving digestion, here are some of the most common essential oils that you might want to have handy at home:

- **Peppermint**

The fresh scent of this essential oil can do more than just give you better breath. If used correctly, it can also help with relieving nausea as well as digestive issues. If you're itching all over and have overworked muscles, it can help in relaxing that too. Congested? Simply add a few drops of it to a bowl of hot water and breathe in the vapor. It should help unclog your airways and make you feel more relaxed.

Peppermint is also great for relieving PMS as well as headaches-- even severe migraines. Another thing it can be used for? - Increasing your focus and concentration. So instead of going for coffee, try some peppermint instead.

- **Lavender**

This is one of the most popular essential oils currently available. It is used in a variety of different ways and products such as perfumes, soaps, lotions and even shampoos! Lavender's popularity is largely attributed to the fact that it is most effective when it comes to calming down the mind and relaxing the body. So if you're tired out after a long day at work, meditating or enjoying the rest of your evening while basking in the scent of lavender oil is certainly something to look forward to.

However, that's not the only thing that this essential oil is capable of providing. High quality lavender oil can be handy in your first aid kit too. It has potent antibacterial properties which are effective when it comes to killing off germs and can easily be used as a substitute for rubbing alcohol. It can also be used as a cleaning product for different areas in your home such as pet cages or even your children's play area. Because of the fact that it is all natural and contains no toxic fumes, you don't need to worry about it affecting your loved one's health.

Other health benefits include: lowers blood pressure, improves sleep quality, relieves joint pain, helps prevent respiratory problems and urinary disorders.

– **Sesame**

Though it is better known for its highly moisturizing qualities, which makes it a favorite when it comes to hair as well as skin treatments, sesame oil's benefits goes way beyond all of that. In fact, it has recently been shown that it can be quite helpful when it comes to slowing down the development of cancer in cells. It is also great for lowering blood pressure and is often used as a substitute for the average vegetable oil. You can easily add it to any salad as a dressing without needing to worry about your heart's overall health. Of course, with that said, do remember to practice moderation when consuming it.

– **Chamomile**

Known to keep insects at bay, it can also help treat a number of different ailments such as: allergies, boils, cuts, arthritis, dermatitis, earache, PMS symptoms, insect bites, headaches, insomnia and sprains. Use it as a massage oil or simply bask in its steam, chamomile oil is always great to have handy because of its numerous uses and benefits.

– **Rose**

When it comes to using rose essential oil, one important consideration that you shouldn't overlook would be getting the highest quality. Look for ones labeled as Rose Otto. The finest ones are produced in Turkey and Bulgaria so if you're really looking to invest a bit of money, these are some of the things you should remember.

Now, quite unlike the oils used for perfumes, this will not carry the same strong scent. Aromatherapists have given it a nickname, "the ultimate woman's oil". This is because of its reputation when it comes to improving hormonal imbalance, treating menopause and PMS symptoms. It can also help with any issues you have in the bedroom-- all while improving both the health and appearance of your skin.

– **Geranium**

This is another great oil for relieving PMS symptoms, but that is not the only purpose it's well suited for. It also contains potent astringent properties which can effectively refresh the skin as well as calm any inflammation and prevent hemorrhaging. Geranium oil is a favorite when it comes to treating acne, both normal and severe cases. Because of the fact that it's all natural, side effects are minimized. It can also help in decreasing facial bloating, boosts circulation in the skin and aids in improving oily skin.

– **Pine**

Though it mostly brings to mind the vision of Christmas trees or simply being in the outdoors, Pine essential oils can do more than just relax the mind. In fact, it is a potent antiseptic, analgesic and antibacterial which makes it a favorite among many holistic health experts. After all, you can use it in three different ways. Often, it is used as a treatment for different skin related issues such as eczema, pimples and psoriasis. However, it can also be used to boost one's metabolism, as an effective antidote for accidental food poisoning, as a treatment for relieving the pain of arthritis and joint pains, for disinfecting wounds and for eliminating respiratory problems that often come about during colder months.

– **Clove**

This is one of the main ingredients used in Tiger Balm, a popular natural remedy that is effective when it comes to relieving hangover headaches. However, that's just one purpose for it. Many holistic health buffs also use it for dental issues such as gum and tooth pain. Some sites even suggest using it for bad breath, though this might not be the best idea unless you're looking for clove-smelling breath.

Clove essential oil is a very potent antiseptic and much like all the other essential oils in this list, you will need to dilute it before using. Once you have the right amount, it can be used as a treatment for scrapes, cuts and bug bites. It can also be used for treating earaches, nasal congestion, digestion problems and stomachaches. Lastly, it is also a known aphrodisiac-- capable of relaxing the mind and removing tension in the muscles.

– **Lemon Balm**

Also known as Melissa essential oil, it may not look like much but it certainly packs quite the punch when it comes to benefits. It is among the most effective and all natural anti-depressants. Along with that, it can also help in keeping your nervous system healthy and working well. It is capable of calming down your anxiety and any inflammation that may or may not be related to it. If you've been experiencing insomnia, this should help you fall asleep easier and deeper. The lemon balm can also help in healing ulcers while fighting any bacterial infections such as herpes. Lastly, it can also help in relieving headaches and lowering your blood pressure.

– **Tea Tree**

While it isn't the most aromatic essential oil available, it certainly has more of a medicinal aroma when compared to others, it is one of the best ones when it comes to treating a number of different ailments. It is also one of the few essential oils that you can use on your skin undiluted - practicing some caution and moderation, of course. Less is certainly more in this case.

Common uses for it include: treatment of candida, acne, chicken pox, cuts, cold sores, insect bites, migraines, flu, sinusitis, warts, oily skin, ring worm and whooping cough.

– **Cinnamon**

Certainly spicy and richer in aroma than most, it is often used as fragrance for candles or even lotions. It gives off a lovely earthy yet bright aroma, often woodsy and slightly peppery. A favorite during colder months because of the warmth it can give off. Some of its most common uses include treatment of: low blood pressure, exhaustion, stress, rheumatism, constipation and scabies.

Chapter 4: How To Use Essential Oils

– Inhalation

This is the most common way of using essential oils and is also connected directly with aromatherapy. Oils can be applied to hot compresses, diffusers or even plain hot water so you can inhale the steam. The standard dose for this method would be 10 drops and is best used for healing respiratory issues, clearing sinuses and relieving headaches. With that said, however, if you inhale highly concentrated essential oils for far too long, this can also cause lethargy, vertigo, nausea and dizziness so do limit your use.

– Baths

When using essential oils for baths, it would be best to mix them with salts first or even an emulsifier such as sesame oil or your favorite bath milk. Aromatic bath salts help in better dispersing the oil into the water while your chosen emulsifier helps it mix into the bath easier. The thing with essential oils, especially if they are concentrated, is that you can't directly add them into water because they won't mix with it and simply end up floating on the surface.

If using essential oils with your bathwater, do avoid the spicier ones, those that you know you're allergic to and phototoxic varieties such as citruses.

– Facial Steam

Just add 1 to 5 drops of the oil into a basin or pot of hot water then cover your head with a towel. Allow the steam to rise and cover your face while breathing normally. Not only is this great for blocked sinuses or awful headaches, it is also wonderful for your skin. You'll feel refreshed right after.

– Massages

Pure essential oils are about 70% more concentrated when compared to the actual plant and as such, carrier oil is required when using one for massages. Now, to make sure you have the proper ratio for this, check the essential oil bottle. Manufacturers always include instructions for diluting the product before using it and applying it onto the skin. Never apply essential oils directly onto your skin as doing so can cause severe allergic reactions, even if you're not allergic to the plant itself. The best carrier oils for this purpose include: olive, sesame and any type of natural nut butters that you prefer.

– Diffusers

This refers to heat resistant vessels that hold your essential oil and basically heat it in order to release its scent. There are many different options available in the market for this depending on the kind that you like. The most common ones are the candle diffuser which uses heat from a candle. This is great if you're looking for light background fragrance. It cannot produce concentrated scents which are what's needed for you to receive therapeutic benefits. Electric heat diffusers are more capable of diffusing thicker oils and can produce very concentrated smells. However, the high heat can actually damage the aromatic compounds if you're not careful.

<u>Important Safety Precautions:</u>

- Never use essential oils internally.

- Never apply it directly onto your skin.

- Keep the bottles out of reach of children.

- Avoid getting it into your eyes.

- Never use citrus oils if you'll be going out into the sun.

- Only use pure essential oils and avoid the ones that contain synthetic fragrances as much as possible. These might be more affordable but the effect isn't the same.

- Never use essential oils on infants, young children, elderly folk, pregnant women and those who have serious health problems.

- Avoid exposing yourself too much to the essential oils without proper ventilation. It can make you dizzy.

- Store the oils properly to avoid rancidity.

Blending Essential Oils:

If you're considering making your own essential oil blends, these are a few of the things that you need to remember:

- Take note of the oil's chemistry. This determines its viscosity, volatility and of course, its properties. These are things that you need to be mindful of when mixing two or three oils together as it can easily affect the outcome.

- The desired action. If you do manage to blend together your oils correctly, it should create a synergistic effect. What this means is that the oil's therapeutic benefits is increased through the mix.

- The sequence of the blend. Lastly, the order in which you blended the essential oils can also be a factor when it comes to the resulting product. Changing this can actually affect its properties as well as the fragrance you produce. Play around with this a bit and see which sequence works well for what you want.

Now, there are also a few rules of thumb that you need to remember when mixing. There isn't much, but knowing these can save you a whole lot of trouble.

- Lighter and smaller molecules will create thinner oils; ones that are less viscous but are more aromatic. They are easily absorbed and are also metabolized much quicker.

- The heavier and larger the molecules are, the thicker the oils they produce but these tend to be less aromatic as well. These kinds of oils don't have a high rate of absorption level, thus, they are metabolized slower.

So why do these things matter?

Well, when you're blending one of each variety together, it can actually make the lighter molecules last longer - meaning, it helps slow down the metabolization process. This is the same principle applied when it comes to perfume making in order to extend the life of the more volatile oils. If you take this and apply it to carrier oils and essential oils, you can create the same kind of effect. This can also be done with two essential oils, you just need to find the best types to mix together. Once you have your essential oil mix, it is also possible to dilute this with carrier oil so that you can use it for aromatherapy massages.

If you're mixing them for that purpose then being mindful of the aroma you produce is of importance. You don't want the oil to end up becoming too aromatic or it may not produce the effect that you want; instead, it could become too much and actually cause dizziness on the part of the person using it. Again, a bit of experimentation is needed on your part in order to get the right blend. Just remember to store your creation properly to make sure that they last long and don't turn rancid in storage.

Chapter 5: Reminders For Purchasing Essential Oils

If it's your first time buying high grade essential oils, there are a few things that you need to keep in mind in order to get the best ones for yourself. Check out the list below:

– Pure

Just because it says "pure" on the label, it doesn't mean that it is. In the US, the term itself does not carry any legal meaning and can be applied to just about anything.

– Synthetic Fragrances

You can easily tell which these ones are. There are certain oil varieties that do not exist in what we often refer to as a "natural state" and can only be bought as bouqueted (synthetic) fragrances which are basically a combination of absolutes, essential oils and a few other synthetic ingredients. Good examples of these would include: gardenia, honeysuckle, frangipani and linden.

– Adulteration

The more expensive a particular essential oil is, the higher the risk of adulteration. Some can be highly adulterated; varieties such as sandalwood, rose and lemon balm are just some of the best examples for this. Then there's also the chain of supply. The more levels are involved in the production of an essential oil, it is more likely that it has been adulterated. It is always best to get your product directly from the distiller, making sure that they use green methods for producing it.

– Extenders

There are oils that are extended using natural solvents - even synthetic ones depending on the manufacturer. The more expensive variety are often extended with natural ones such as jojoba.

– Container

There are vendors who actually sell their products in aluminum containers instead of using tinted bottles. It has been said that aluminum can affect the quality of the oil because it may cause a chemical reaction. This type of container is only acceptable if the inside has been lined. Another consideration is to avoid buying ones with a rubber eyedropper bulb on top. High quality essential oils can actually dissolve the rubber and then become contaminated by it.

– FDA Regulations

If you're going to be purchasing essential oils a lot and want to be sure of the ones you're getting, then familiarizing yourself with the FDA regulations will educate you on which things are acceptable and which ones aren't.

– Choose Organic

This one's a no-brainer. Organic products are going to be superior when compared to non-organic oils; not to mention the fact that it is safer to use as well.

– Ask For Samples

While some vendors may be hesitant in providing this, asking for a sample will actually allow you to better ascertain the quality of the product. However, don't ask for a sample of everything. Go for 2 to 4 samples of the ones you're sincerely interested in purchasing. Some vendors do offer sample sized bottles for a price and while shelling out some cash for a small amount of product isn't exactly appealing, it still is a good option if you really want to try the oils out before committing to buying them.

Chapter 6: Carrier Oils And Essential Oils

If you're planning on using essential oils often then you need to familiarize yourself with carrier oils and their purpose.

– *What are carrier oils?*

These are oils that are derived from the fattier portion of plants, usually from the seeds, nuts and kernels of it. Carrier oils are also often used to dilute essential oils prior to using it topically. This is where it gets its name from as well; given that their purpose is to "carry" the essential oil onto the skin. However, this is not the only thing that carrier oils are useful for. They too can offer different therapeutic benefits and contain many vitamins, minerals as well as essential fatty acids which are all great for improving the skin. Carrier oils are also capable of treating different conditions such as psoriasis and eczema. For beauty purposes, they can help reduce wrinkles as well as the appearance of scar tissue. In fact, they are also often used as a way to diminish acne scars.

Natural body lotions, creams, bath oils, body oils, lip balm and other skin care products that are meant to moisturize also often make use of carrier oils. It can affect the scent, color, therapeutic benefits and even the shelf life of the product itself.

Technically, they are classified as fixed oils because they do not evaporate unlike some. They are also, as we've mentioned earlier, typically derived from seeds and nuts though there are a few exceptions to this. For example, the coconut oil is derived from the white flesh known as copra through a special process. Jojoba oil is actually not an oil but a liquid wax that's derived from the leathery-leaved shrub. It is also one of the most commonly used ones especially when it comes to body lotions, creams and butters.

    — *Choosing a carrier oil to use*

There are a wide range of carrier oils to choose from and it all depends on what your need and purpose for it is. All you really have to know are a few basic facts when it comes to properties, viscosity and actions-- all of which provide you with the information you need in order to choose the best kind.

Because of the fact that it is typically used as a skin treatment, choosing the finest oils is the best thing to do. However, compared to your average carrier or base oil, these are also a bit more expensive. If you're using it for aromatherapy, experimenting with oil mixes until you find what works best for you is a good option to try.

- What are some of the best carrier oil varieties?

When it comes to versatility, peach, sweet almond and apricot can be used for both body massages as well as facial treatments. This is because of the fact that they are lighter than other varieties and are easily absorbed by the skin. For those who are a tad worried about getting an allergic reaction from nut oils then opting for Sunflower is a great alternative.

Other oils you can use for facial treatments, which can also be mixed with your favorite essential oil, include: Rosehip, Jojoba, Borage, Black Seed and Evening Primrose. They might need a bit of diluting for use as a massage oil but they certainly deliver when it comes to facial purposes. You can also try Wheatgerm and unrefined avocado as an overnight treatment when it comes to nourishing your skin. While they do have a significantly strong odor, once you get past it, they can provide you with excellent nourishing oils that will soften and give your skin a youthful feel.

So the next time you're choosing a carrier oil for your needs, consider the above things!

Conclusion

Thank you again for downloading this book!

I hope this book was able to help you learn more about aromatherapy!

The next step is to put this information to use, and begin using aromatherapy and essential oils at home!

Finally, if you enjoyed this book, please take the time to share your thoughts and post a review on Amazon. It'd be greatly appreciated!

Thank you and good luck!